Mediterranean Delights Cookbook

A Collection of Delicious Mediterranean Recipes for Healthy & Tasty Meals

Marta Jackson

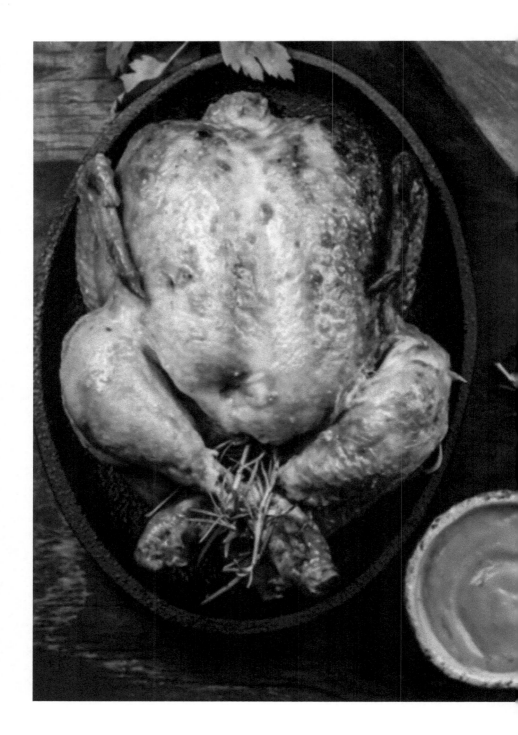

By reading this document, the reader agrees that under no circumstances is the author responsible for any losses, direct or indirect, which are incurred as a result of the use of information contained within this document, including, but not limited to, — errors, omissions, or inaccuracies.

Table of Contents

Creamed spinach

Ingredients

- 100g of cheddar cheese
- 2 onions
- 100g of unsalted butter
- 2 cloves of garlic
- 100g of plain flour
- Olive oil
- 2 teaspoons of dried oregano
- 250ml crème fraiche
- 1 whole nutmeg
- 1kg of frozen chopped spinach
- 100g of rolled oats

Directions

- Preheat the oven to 350°F.
- Place onions and garlic, oregano, and 2 tablespoons of olive oil in a large frying pan on a low heat.
- Grate in half of the nutmeg, fry for 10 minutes, or until soft, stirring regularly.

- Add the spinach, raise the heat to medium, let cook for 20 minutes, or until any liquid has evaporated.
- Place butter with cheese flour, oats, and a pinch of sea salt and black pepper in a blender.
- Blend into a crumble texture, then remove to a plate.
- Put the cooked spinach mixture into the processor, then add the crème fraiche, blend for 1 minute.
- Taste, and adjust the seasoning.
- Place evenly into a baking dish.
- Sprinkle over the crumble, let bake for around 45 minutes, or until golden.
- Serve and enjoy.

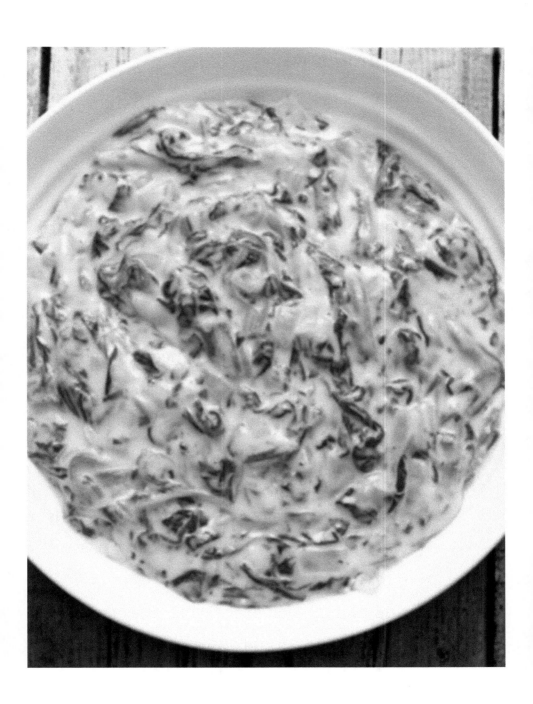

Speedy spinach curry

Ingredients

- 100g of paneer cheese
- 20g of unsalted cashew nuts
- 200g of baby spinach
- 1 onion
- Red wine vinegar
- 2 teaspoons of Rogan curry paste

Directions

- Put a large frying pan on a medium-high heat.
- Toast the cashew nuts as it heats up, shaking the pan occasionally until lightly golden.
- Place the cashews into a pestle and mortar, returning the pan to the heat.
- Place sliced onion in the hot pan with 1 tablespoon of olive oil and the curry paste.
- Cook and stir for 8 minutes.
- Add 1 tablespoon of red wine vinegar.
- Let the vinegar cook away briefly, then, dice and add the paneer followed by the spinach.

- Stir until the spinach is wilted, and liquid evaporated
- Season with sea salt and black pepper.
- Crush the cashew nuts and sprinkle over the top.
- Serve and enjoy.

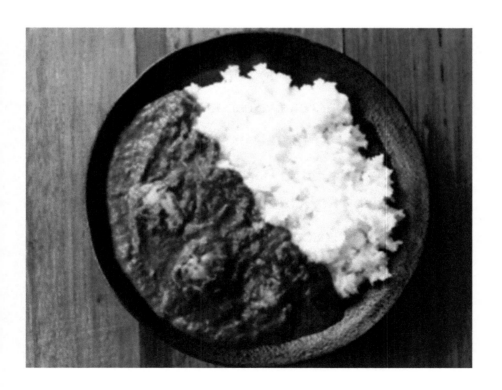

Smoky pancetta cod

Ingredients

- 1 x 250g sachet of cooked lentils
- 200g of spinach
- Red wine vinegar
- 8 rashers of smoked pancetta
- 2 x 150g of white fish fillets
- 2 sprigs of fresh rosemary

Directions

- Lay out 4 rashers of pancetta, slightly overlapping them.
- Place a piece of cod on top.
- Then, generously season with black pepper.
- Roll and wrap in the pancetta, and repeat.
- Place in a large frying pan on a medium heat, let cook for 8 minutes, turning occasionally.
- Add the rosemary for the last 2 minutes.
- Remove the fish to a plate.
- Toss the lentils into the pan with 1 tablespoon of red wine vinegar and push to one side to reheat for 1 minute.

- Taste, and adjust the seasoning with sea salt and pepper
- Sit the wrapped cod on top of the lentils with the rosemary.
- Drizzle with 1 teaspoon of extra virgin olive oil.
- Serve and enjoy.

Wilted spinach with yogurt and raisins

Ingredients

- 40g of raisins
- Extra virgin olive oil
- 1 small clove of garlic
- 300g of frozen spinach
- 500g of Greek yoghurt
- Sunflower oil

Directions

- Place the spinach in a saucepan with a few tablespoons of water and cook over a medium heat briefly, or until defrosted.
- Let cool.
- Mix crushed garlic with the yoghurt, ¾ of a teaspoon of sea salt and a generous grind of black pepper.
- Stir in the cooled spinach.
- Heat sunflower oil in a small pan and fry the raisins for 2 minutes.
- Scatter over the spinach and finish with a drizzle of extra virgin olive oil.

- Serve and enjoy.

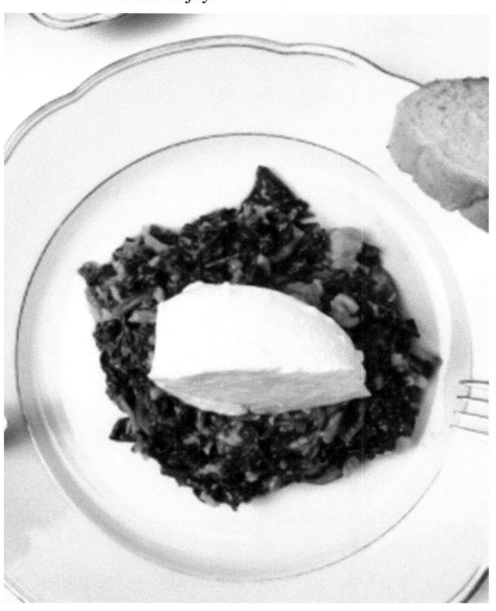

Spinach pici pasta

Ingredients

- Olive oil
- Extra virgin olive oil
- 4 cloves of garlic
- 50g of Parmesan cheese
- ½ teaspoon of dried red chili flakes
- 200g of baby spinach
- ½ a bunch of fresh basil
- 200g of baby courgettes
- 300g of plain flour
- 320g of ripe cherry tomatoes
- 50g of pine nuts

Directions

- In a food processor, blend the spinach with flour until a ball of dough forms.
- Tear off balls of dough, roll them out into long thin sausage shapes.
- Cook the pici immediately, or leave them to dry out for a few hours.
- Put a large pan of salted water to boil.

- Put a large frying pan on a medium heat with 2 tablespoons of olive oil.
- Add the sliced garlic with the chili flakes.
- Add the courgettes with halved tomatoes, let cook for 5 minutes.
- Stir in the pine nuts with a ladleful of boiling water. Cook over low heat.
- Add the pici to the pan of boiling salted water for 8 5 minutes, and 8 minutes for dry one.
- Drain, reserving a mugful of cooking water, toss through the vegetables.
- Reserving the baby basil leaves, Stir into the pan the big chopped ones with grated Parmesan.
- Divide between warm plates and serve with a few drips of extra virgin olive oil.
- Enjoy.

Spinach lasagna

Ingredients

- 50g of plain flour
- 300g of fresh lasagna sheets
- 800ml of milk
- 100g of Parmesan cheese
- 1 fresh bay leaf
- 70g of unsalted butter
- 1 whole nutmeg
- 800g of spinach
- 200g of ricotta cheese

Directions

- Preheat the oven ready to 375°F.
- Melt the butter in a pan, then whisk in the flour.
- Cook for 2 minutes, whisk in the milk till smooth.
- Season with sea salt and freshly ground black pepper.
- Add the bay leaf, let simmer for 5 minutes. Turn off the heat.

- Remove the stalks from the spinach, then wilt with the remaining 20g butter in a covered pan, drain, let cool and squeeze out the liquid.
- Mix chopped spinach with the ricotta and a ladleful of the white sauce and nutmeg. Season.
- In a baking dish, layer the lasagna sheets with white sauce, spinach mixture, and a grating of Parmesan.
- Finish with a layer of pasta topped with sauce and more Parmesan.
- Let bake for 30 minutes, or till golden.
- Serve and enjoy.

Monkfish with spinach and feta

Ingredients

- 50g of feta cheese
- 1 teaspoon of cumin seeds
- 200g of spinach
- ½ of a lemon
- 2 x 150g of monkfish fillets
- 2 sprigs of fresh thyme
- Olive oil

Directions

- Crush and sprinkle the cumin seeds over the monkfish fillets.
- Sprinkle the thyme leaves on top and season well.
- Heat a little olive oil over a medium heat.
- Add the fish and fry for 4 minutes on each side.
- Bring a large pan of salted water to the boil.
- Then, blanch the spinach for about 3 minutes.
- Drain and drizzle with oil.
- Serve and enjoy with the monkfish, sprinkled with the feta.

Spring pie

Ingredients

- 1 lemon
- Olive oil
- 1 x 270g packet of filo pastry
- 1 teaspoon of mustard powder
- 3 medium leeks
- 200ml of milk
- 200g of baby spinach
- 6 rashers of smoked streaky bacon
- ½ a bunch of fresh chives
- 6 large free-range eggs

Directions

- Start by preheating the oven ready to 350°F.
- Grease the baking dish with olive oil.
- Cover the baking dish with a layer of pastry, letting the edges overhang slightly.
- Brush with bit of olive oil.
- Add another layer of pastry, repeating until all the pastry is done

- Boil the kettle, then place the spinach in a colander.
- Pour over the hot water to wilt.
- Push the spinach down with the back of a spoon, then, when it's cool enough to handle, squeeze out any excess water.
- Place the spinach on a board and roughly chop, then place in a large bowl and set aside.
- Put the grill on high and grill the bacon till crisp, let cool.
- Whisk the eggs in a large bowl with a pinch of sea salt and black pepper.
- Then, whisk in the milk together with the mustard powder, chives, and grate in the lemon zest.
- Crumble the cooled bacon into the spinach.
- Add the leeks. Mix and scatter into the filo pastry case.
- Pour over the egg mixture and place the dish on the bottom of the oven.
- Let bake for 40 minutes.
- Let cool for 20 minutes.

- Serve sliced and enjoy with a crisp green salad.

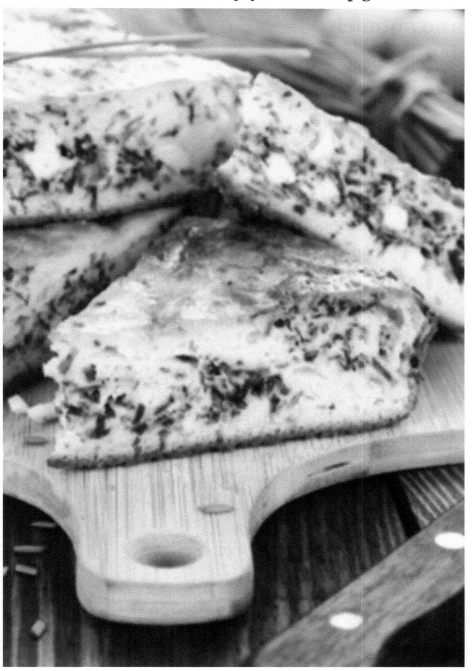

Curried cauliflower, potatoes, chickpeas, and spinach

Ingredients

- 1 teaspoon of ground cumin
- 1 cauliflower
- 1 teaspoon of mustard seeds
- 800g of potatoes
- 1 teaspoon of ground ginger
- 2 cloves of garlic
- Natural yoghurt
- 1 teaspoon of ground coriander
- 1 onion
- 1 teaspoon of curry powder
- 1 long green chili
- 2 tablespoons of olive oil
- 2 tablespoons of unsalted butter
- 1 lime
- 1 teaspoon of turmeric
- 1 x 400g tin of chickpeas
- 250g of baby spinach

Directions

- Cook separated cauliflower in boiling salted water for 5 minutes, drain, reserve some of its cooking water.
- Roughly chop the potatoes and cook in boiling salted water for 10 minutes, drain excess water.
- Heat the olive oil and butter in a large frying pan, then sauté the garlic with the onion and chili till softened over low heat.
- Stir in all the spices.
- Season, let cook briefly.
- Add the cooked cauliflower, potatoes, and reserved cooking water.
- Let simmer over low heat for 10 minutes.
- Drain and add the chickpeas with the spinach.
- Cook, stirring, until the spinach wilts.
- Then, transfer to a serving bowl.
- Serve and enjoy with a dollop of yoghurt and a squeeze of lime juice.

Healthy greens box

Ingredients

- 1 heaped teaspoon harissa
- ½ a small head of broccoli
- 50g of feta cheese
- 1 handful of mixed seeds
- 1 handful of baby spinach
- ½ a small bunch of fresh mint
- Olive oil
- 80g of couscous
- 1 lemon
- 1 pinch of ground cumin

Directions

- Cook the chopped broccoli in boiling water for 4 minutes.
- Plunge into cold water to stop it cooking, then shake off excess water, place on a chopping board with the spinach.
- Pick over a few large mint leaves and throw on a good pinch of salt and pepper.
- Chop until finely chopped.

- Scrape these straight into your lunchbox, pour the uncooked couscous on top and gently sit a lemon half in it.
- Toast the seeds in a dry frying pan, then mix with the cumin and wrap in Clingfilm.
- Add the juice from the remaining lemon half with a good swig of olive oil, harissa, and a few small mint leaves, then crumble in the feta in a small jar. Mix well.
- Seal and place in the lunch box.
- Boil the kettle when it is time to feast.
- Take the lemon, seeds and jar from your lunchbox, then pour in boiling water to just cover the couscous.
- Cover, and wait for 10 minutes until the water is absorbed.
- Serve and enjoy.

Brilliant broccoli

Ingredients

- A small knob of unsalted butter
- 1 large head of broccoli
- Sea salt
- Freshly ground black pepper

Directions

- Fill a large pan with slightly salted water, bring to the boil over a high heat.
- Once boiling, lower the broccoli into the water using a slotted spoon.
- Let cook for 4 minutes.
- Drain in a colander, steam dry for a minute.
- Place back into the pan, sprinkle with a tiny pinch of salt and pepper.
- Add the butter tossing to coat.
- Serve and enjoy.

Steamed vegetables with flavored butters

Ingredients

- 500g of baby turnips
- 1 pinch of cumin seeds
- 350g of broccoli, cut into florets
- 1 tablespoon of fresh thyme
- Unsalted butter
- 1 clove garlic, chopped
- 450g of carrots, cut into thick strips
- 1 pinch of sugar
- ¼ orange, finely grated zest of
- ½ tablespoon of chopped fresh rosemary
- 3 anchovy fillets, chopped
- 2 sun-dried tomatoes in oil, drained and finely chopped
- ½ lemon
- 350g of mange tout, trimmed
- ½ red chili, deseeded and finely chopped

Directions

- Pound the garlic together with the chili and sun-dried tomatoes in a pestle and mortar to a paste.
- Add seasoning and the butter, pound well.
- Dollop onto a sheet of greaseproof paper and roll into a cylinder, twisting the ends.
- Place in the freezer to firm up.
- Then, pound the sugar together with the zest, cumin seeds, and thyme.
- Combine the broccoli, the rosemary, and anchovies, pound.
- Mix the lemon juice and zest.
- Then add the seasoning and butter, pound and roll into Christmas cracker shapes, as before.
- Place the vegetables in a 2-layer steamer. Make sure carrots are closer to the heat, turnips, broccoli florets, then mange tout.
- Steam for 10 minutes.
- Serve and enjoy each vegetable with circles of flavored butter melted over the top.

Broccoli salad

Ingredients

- 6 tablespoons of extra virgin olive oil
- 2 large heads of broccoli
- 2 teaspoons of Dijon mustard
- 6 rashers of smoked streaky bacon
- 3 firm red tomatoes
- 2 tablespoons of white wine vinegar
- Olive oil
- ½ a bunch of fresh chives
- ½ a clove of garlic

Directions

- Blanch the broccoli florets and sliced stalks quickly in boiling salted water for 60 seconds.
- Drain in a colander, steam dry.
- Transfer to a serving dish once totally dry.
- Then, fry the sliced bacon on a medium heat with a small splash of olive oil until crisp and golden.
- Spoon most of the bacon bits over the broccoli.

- Pour into a mixing bowl, then grate in the garlic, adding the Dijon mustard, extra virgin olive oil, white wine vinegar.
- Season with sea salt and black pepper, and whisk.
- Chop the chives, reserving the flowers.
- Add to the broccoli and bacon bits.
- Serve and enjoy.

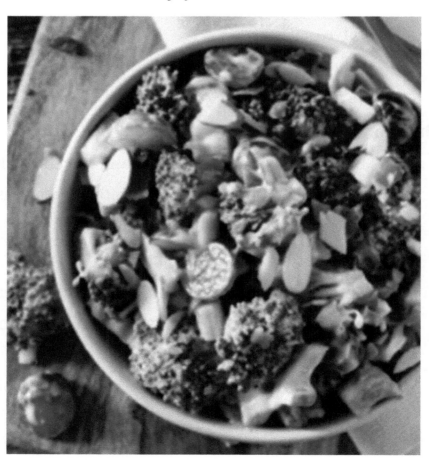

Mango, spinach, and pine nuts recipe

Ingredients

- ½ of a ripe mango
- 1 large handful of baby spinach
- 2 tablespoons of Greek yoghurt
- 1 tablespoon of pine nuts

Directions

- Prepare the mangoes into bite-sized chunks.
- Place in a blender.
- Add the yoghurt together with the spinach and pine nuts, blend to a purée.
- Adjust the thickness with water to loosen.
- Serve and enjoy chilled.

Sag paneer

Ingredients

- freshly ground black pepper
- groundnut oil
- 1 onion
- 1.5 liters of whole milk
- 2 cloves of garlic
- 600g of frozen spinach
- 5cm piece of ginger
- 1 lemon
- sea salt
- 1 teaspoon of cumin seeds
- 2 teaspoons of Garam masala
- 50ml of single cream
- ½ teaspoon of ground turmeric
- 1 ripe tomato

Directions

- Line a sieve with a large piece of muslin and place over a bowl.
- Heat the milk in a large heavy-based pan over a medium heat.

- Bring to the boil, then reduce the heat to a gentle simmer.
- Add 4 tablespoons of lemon juice, then pour the mixture into the sieve. Place under cold running water, gather up the muslin and squeeze out the excess moisture.
- Place in the fridge for 1 hour 30 minutes, then cut the paneer into chunks.
- Drizzle olive oil into a large non-stick frying pan over a medium heat, place in the paneer and fry for 5 minutes, stirring frequently. Drain.
- Return the pan to a medium-low heat, add cumin seeds and onion, fry for 8 minute, or until softened.
- Stir in the garlic with ginger, Garam masala, chopped tomatoes, and turmeric. Cook for 10 minutes, stirring occasionally.
- Stir in the frozen spinach, then add the cream, paneer and a splash of boiling water.

- Lower the heat, let cook for 5 minutes uncovered, or until reduced to a creamy consistency.
- Season with sea salt and black pepper.
- Serve and enjoy.

Chickpea and spiced spinach smash with sweet potato

Ingredients

- 1 x 400g tin of chickpeas in water
- 1 teaspoon of olive oil
- 1 small onion
- 200g of fresh spinach
- 1 clove of garlic
- 1 large sweet potato
- ½ teaspoon of garam masala
- ½ teaspoon of turmeric

Directions

- Cook the sweet potato in boiling water until tender, drain and mash.
- Heat the oil in a medium pan over low heat.
- Add the onion and fry for 8 minutes.
- Add the garlic together with the turmeric and garam masala, cook for 3 minutes.
- Drain the chickpeas, add to the pan along with the spinach.

- Cover, let cook for 10 minutes, or until the spinach has wilted.
- Mash the mixture with until fairly smooth with some soft lumps, let cool.
- Serve the cooled chickpea smash with the mashed sweet potato.
- Enjoy.

Gluten-free spinach and ricotta roulade

Ingredients

- Olive oil
- 1 lemon
- 1 pinch of chili flakes
- 2 cloves of garlic
- 60g of whole blanched almonds
- 1 fresh red chili
- 1 kg butternut squash
- 1 teaspoon of fennel seeds
- 6 large free-range eggs
- 100g of crumbly goat's cheese
- 80g of Parmesan cheese
- 150g of ricotta cheese
- 60g of gluten-free plain flour
- 1 whole nutmeg
- 300g of baby spinach

Directions

- Preheat the oven to 375°F.
- Line a shallow baking tin with greaseproof paper.

- Place prepared squash into a large roasting tray with a splash of olive oil, chili flakes, and bit of pinch of salt and pepper. Toss to coat.
- Add garlic cloves, then place in the hot oven for 1 hour.
- Place a frying pan over a medium heat with almonds, fennel seeds, and a pinch of salt.
- Let cook for 4 minutes, or until golden. Bash in a mortar.
- Remove from oven, then scoop the flesh and garlic into a food processor and discard the skin. Blend till smooth.
- Separate the egg yolks from the whites into two large bowls.
- Grate the Parmesan over the yolks, stir in the squash purée together with the flour, nutmeg, and a pinch of salt and pepper.
- Fold into the squash mixture.
- Transfer to the lined tin, spreading evenly.
- Let bake for 15 minutes, or until set.

- Heat a splash of olive oil over a medium heat, add spinach, let cook for 2 minutes until wilted.
- Turn out the roulade onto a large piece of greaseproof paper.
- Crumble the goat's cheese into a bowl, add the ricotta together with the lemon zest and juice.
- Add chili, stir.
- Season with sea salt and black pepper.
- Spread the mixture over the sponge, scatter over the spinach and 1/3 of the almonds.
- Roll up the sponge, using the greaseproof paper.
- Serve and enjoy.

Giant vegetable rosti

Ingredients

- 100g of baby spinach
- 600g of potatoes
- 3 large carrots
- Olive oil
- 4 large free-range eggs
- 100g of frozen peas
- ½ teaspoon of Dijon mustard
- 50g of feta cheese
- ½ of a lemon
- Extra virgin olive oil

Directions

- Preheat the oven to 350°F.
- Coarsely grate potatoes and carrots in a food processor.
- Add a good pinch of sea salt, toss, let rest for 5 minutes.
- Combine the mustard together with a squeeze of lemon juice, extra virgin olive oil, and a little

pinch of salt and black pepper in a medium bowl.

- Drizzle olive oil into a large bowl.
- Add a good pinch of pepper.
- Then, squeeze the potato and carrot mixture, then sprinkle into the bowl.
- Toss in the oil with the pepper until mixed.
- Scatter over a large oiled baking tray.
- Roast for 35 minutes or so, until golden on top.
- In a large pan of salted boiling water, blanch the peas for a minute.
- Then, add to the bowl of dressing and pile the spinach on top.
- Crack in the eggs when the rosti is about to get ready, poach and remove.
- Serve the rosti with the eggs on top.
- Serve and enjoy.

Perfect braised spinach

Ingredients

- 10g of butter
- 400g of spinach
- 1 grating nutmeg
- ½ lemon, juice

Directions

- Place little butter, nutmeg grating, spinach, and a tiny squeeze of lemon juice into a pan.
- Cover, and cook with steam.
- Let the spinach sit for a minute.
- Serve and enjoy.

Roast trout with spinach, sage, and prosciutto

Ingredients

- 410g of tinned cannellini beans
- 75g of ground almonds
- 2 handfuls of dried apricots, chopped
- 4 large slices quality prosciutto
- 2 large sprigs fresh sage
- 600g of spinach
- Olive oil
- 8 x 120g of trout fillets
- 410g of tinned chickpeas
- 1 clove garlic, crushed
- Fresh nutmeg, grated

Directions

- Preheat the oven to 400°F.
- Season the trout with salt and pepper, dust in the ground almonds.
- Lay 4 of the fillets on a board, skin-side down.
- Mix apricot and ½ of the sage together, then lay in a line along the tops of the 4 fillets.

- Top with the remaining fillets, skin-side up, matching heads and tails with the 4 below.
- Overlap the remaining sage along the length of each trout sandwich.
- Cut 4 x 20cm lengths of string and lay them parallel to each other on a work surface.
- Lay 1 of the trout sandwiches across the lengths of string and tie them all up.
- Repeat with the rest.
- Heat a large saucepan.
- Add a large splash of oil and gently fry the garlic until softened.
- Add the spinach, seasoning with salt and pepper and the grated nutmeg.
- Spread the spinach out in a roasting tray, and mix with the pulses.
- Lay the prosciutto slices over the bean mixture.
- Drizzle with olive oil, bake for 20 minutes until the prosciutto is crispy.

Cumberland roast chicken

Ingredients

- 1 x 1.5kg of whole chicken
- 1.2 kg potatoes
- 3 Cumberland sausages
- 1 pear
- 2 parsnips
- 2 leeks
- 85g of watercress
- Olive oil
- ½ bunch of sage

Directions

- Preheat the oven to 360°F.
- Place potatoes, parsnips, and leeks in a roasting tray, then toss with 2 tablespoons of olive oil, a pinch of sea salt and black pepper and the sage leaves.
- Squeeze the sausage meat out of the skins, make sure to scrunch together.
- Poke half the sausage meat into each side, smooth well.

- Secure the skin with a cocktail stick.
- Rub the chicken with a pinch of salt and pepper and 1 tablespoon of oil.
- Stuff the sage stalks into the chicken cavity.
- Place the chicken directly on the bars of the oven with the tray of vegetables underneath, let roast until everything is golden.
- Sprinkle the reserved sage leaves over the tray of vegetables.
- Slice the pear, and toss with the watercress.
- Sit the chicken on the vegetables.
- Serve and enjoy.

Sausage and mash pie

Ingredients

- 6 Cumberland
- 4 tablespoons of plain flour
- Olive oil
- 3 teaspoons of English mustard
- 2 large leeks
- 1.2kg of potatoes
- ½ a bunch of thyme
- 2 eating apples
- 600ml of semi-skimmed milk

Directions

- Preheat the oven to 400°F.
- Cook chopped potatoes in a large pan of salted boiling water for 15 minutes.
- In a large non-stick casserole pan, brown the sausages on a medium heat, tossing regularly.
- Add 1 tablespoon of olive oil with the leek.
- Remove the sausages once golden, place in the leek with apple, thyme, and splash of water.

- Season with sea salt and black pepper, cook for 20 minutes, covered, stirring occasionally.
- Drain the potatoes, and mash with half of the flour.
- Lightly rub a baking dish with oil.
- Spread 2/3 of the mash evenly across the base and sides of the dish.
- Stir the remaining flour into the leeks, together with the milk, and mustard.
- Simmer for 5 minutes.
- Stir sausages into the pan with any juices, then evenly spoon into the mash-lined dish.
- Press the remaining mash on to a sheet of greaseproof paper until bigger than the dish, then flip over the top of the dish, crimp the edges with a fork to seal.
- Poke the reserved sausage slices into the top, brush with 1 tablespoon of oil.
- Let bake for 40 minutes.
- Serve and enjoy.

Sweet leek carbonara

Ingredients

- Olive oil
- 2 large leeks
- 4 cloves of garlic
- 50g of Parmesan or pecorino cheese
- 1 large free-range egg
- 4 sprigs of fresh thyme
- 1 knob of unsalted butter
- 300g of dried spaghetti

Directions

- Combine the leek and garlic in a large casserole pan over medium heat with the butter and 1 tablespoon of olive oil.
- When sizzling, stir in the leeks and water, let simmer, covered over a low heat for 40 minutes, stirring occasionally.
- Season with sea salt and black pepper.
- Then, cook the pasta in a large pan of boiling salted water according to the packet Directions.

- Drain, reserving some pasta cooking water.
- Toss the drained pasta into the leek pan, then remove from the heat.
- Hold on for 2 minutes to let cool briefly, then beat in eggs with cheese, toss.
- Serve and enjoy with white wine.

Quiche leekraine

Ingredients

- 250ml of milk
- 300g of leeks
- 1 x 20cm precooked pastry case
- Olive oil
- 3 large eggs
- 3 slices of smoked streaky bacon
- Green salad
- 75g of Cheddar cheese

Directions

- Preheat the oven to 360°F.
- Sauté the leek with a splash of oil until sticky.
- Fry the chopped bacon in a separate pan until golden.
- Whisk the eggs and stir the cheese in the cheese, milk, leeks, bacon, and pinch of seasoning.
- Place the pastry case onto a baking sheet.
- Pour the mixture into the case.
- Let bake for 30 minutes.

- Serve and enjoy with a mixed green salad.

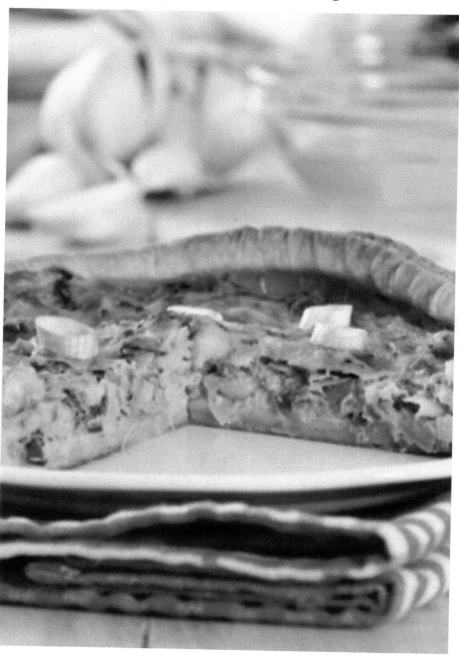

Ham and peas

Ingredients

- ½ a bunch of fresh curly parsley
- 3 ham hocks
- 400g of frozen peas
- 100g of pearl barley
- 2 leeks
- 1 stick of celery
- 1 heaped tablespoon of mint sauce
- 3 carrots
- Olive oil
- 2 fresh bay leaves
- 1 liter of organic chicken stock

Directions

- Soak the ham hocks in cold water overnight.
- Drain, refill with fresh cold water and bring to the boil.
- Discard the salty water, rinse the hocks, repeat once again.
- Combine the leeks with the celery, and carrots in a food processor.

- Add the vegetables to a pan with olive oil, bay leaves, a pinch of sea salt and black pepper.
- Sweat over a medium heat for 15 minutes, stirring occasionally.
- Add the drained ham hocks, pearl barley, and chicken stock.
- Let boil, then cook over a medium-low heat for 3 hours when covered.
- Transfer the ham hocks to a clean board, remove all the fat and bones.
- Shred the meat then return it to the broth.
- Raise the heat, add the peas.
- Cook until tender, then finely chop and stir in the parsley with the mint sauce.
- Serve and enjoy with bread.

Cheesy leeks

Ingredients

- 50g of Parmesan cheese
- 6 large leeks
- 1 knob of unsalted butter
- 2 cloves of garlic
- 100g of Cheddar cheese
- 100g of brie
- 5 sprigs of fresh thyme
- Olive oil
- 100ml of single cream

Directions

- Preheat the oven to 350°F.
- Over a medium heat, place a large casserole pan
- Drizzle with bit of oil, butter, thyme leaves, and garlic.
- Cook until bubbling, fry, then stir in the leeks.
- Stir the rest of the ingredients into the leeks, with grated Cheddar and Parmesan, and brie,

then place in the oven cook for 45 minutes uncovered.

- Season, then spoon it all into a dish.
- Stir in the cream and splash of water.
- Grate over the Cheddar and Parmesan.
- Pull the brie into parts, place on top.
- Place in the oven for 15 minutes.
- Serve and enjoy.

Crostini of smoked salmon butter and poached leeks

Ingredients

- 5 sprigs of fresh chervil
- 160g of unsalted butter
- 200ml of white wine
- 10 baby leeks
- 130g of smoked salmon
- 60g of unsalted butter
- 60ml of olive oil
- 20ml of fresh lemon juice
- 2 fresh bay leaves
- 12 slices of ciabatta
- 3 sprigs of fresh thyme
- 200ml of quality fish stock
- 40g of salted baby capers

Directions

- Combine the butter with smoked salmon, and lemon juice in a food processor, blend until smooth.
- Season and set aside.

- Combine butter, olive oil, bay leaves, and thyme to a wide, shallow saucepan over a medium-low heat, let simmer.
- Add the leeks, let cook for 10 minutes, until golden.
- Pour in the stock with the wine, cover with a baking paper, let cook for 15 minutes.
- Remove from the heat and rest the leeks in the liquid.
- Put the capers in a small saucepan with enough olive oil to cover.
- Place over a high heat, fry until the capers crisp up.
- Transfer the capers to a plate lined with kitchen paper using a slotted spoon.
- Heat a griddle pan over medium high heat.
- Brush the ciabatta with olive oil and toast until golden.
- Spread the toasted ciabatta generously with the smoked salmon butter.
- Serve and enjoy topped with the leeks and fried capers

Ham and leek quiche

Ingredients

- 300ml of semi-skimmed milk
- 2 leeks
- 1 shallot
- 8 sprigs of fresh thyme
- 4 sheets of filo pastry
- 75g of mature Cheddar
- 60g of smoked ham
- 3 large eggs
- 10g of unsalted butter
- 200g of sprouting broccoli
- 1 tablespoon of olive oil

Directions

- Preheat the oven to 350°F.
- Melt butter in a pan, then sauté the leeks with the shallot and half the thyme leaves for 5 minutes.
- Blanch the broccoli in boiling salted water for about 3 minutes. Drain.

- Brush a quiche tin with a little of the olive oil, drape with a layer of filo pastry, leaving some overhanging.
- Brush the filo with a little more oil.
- Scatter over some of the remaining thyme leaves and layer another piece of filo on top. Repeat layering the oil, thyme and filo until you have a fully lined quiche base.
- Bake the case for 5 minutes.
- Stir the broccoli together with the smoked ham through the leek mixture.
- Spoon the filling over the pastry base.
- Beat the eggs with milk and a pinch of black pepper, grate in cheese.
- Pour over the vegetables and ham.
- Place grate over the rest of the cheese.
- Place the baking tray, let bake for 30 minutes.
- Let rest for 15 minutes, serve and enjoy.

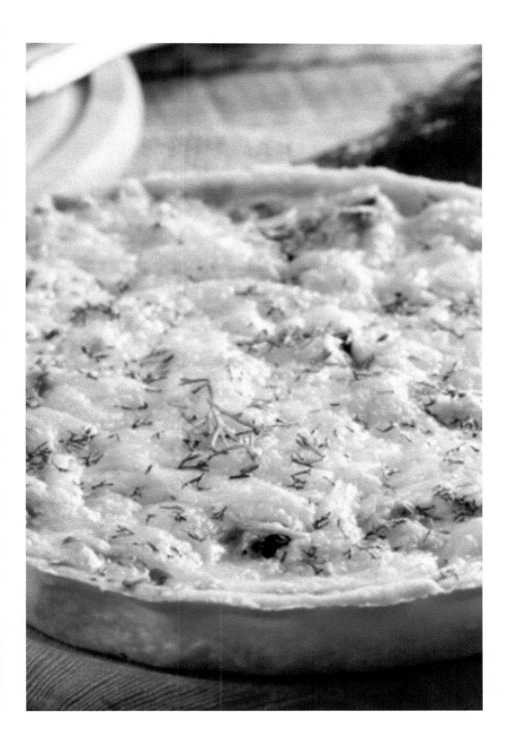

Leek, potato, and pea soup

Ingredients

- A few sprigs of fresh flat-leaf parsley
- 2 large leeks
- 200g of frozen peas
- 1 large potato
- 1½ tablespoons of olive oil
- 1 teaspoon of bouillon powder
- 400ml of milk

Directions

- Begin by heating olive oil over medium heat.
- Then, add the leek together with the potatoes, fry for 5 minutes.
- Add the bouillon powder.
- Pour in 400ml water, reduce the heat, simmer for 10 minutes.
- Add the milk together with the parsley and peas to the pan, simmer for a further 5 minutes to warm through.
- Serve and enjoy.

Chickpea, leek, and carrot stew

Ingredients

- ½ tablespoon of olive oil
- 1 small leek
- 1 small carrot
- 2 tablespoons of natural yoghurt
- 1 x 210g tin of chickpeas

Directions

- Heat olive oil in a medium pan over medium heat.
- Add the leek, let cook until softened, then add the carrots with 200ml water.
- Bring to the boil, when covered, then reduce to a simmer for until the vegetables are tender.
- Drain, then add the chickpeas, let warm through for 5 minutes, then remove.
- Let cool briefly, then stir through the yoghurt.
- Mash until fairly smooth, with some soft lumps.
- Serve and enjoy.

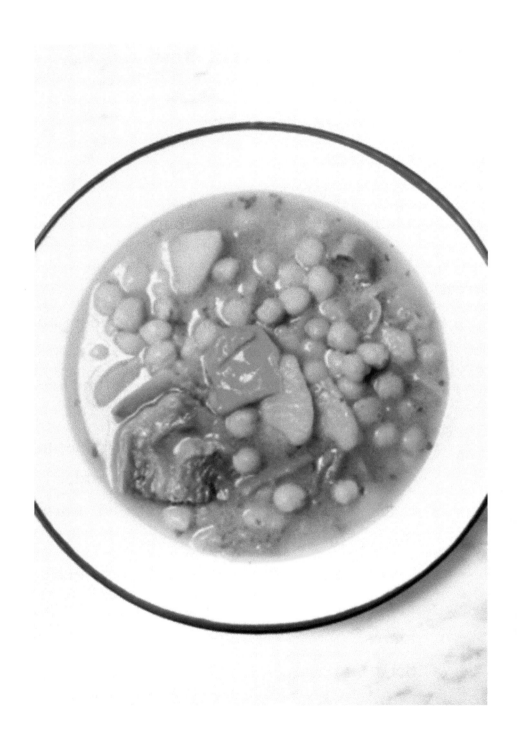

Chicken, leek, and pea pasta bake

Ingredients

- 200g of cooked chicken
- 1 tablespoon butter
- 225ml of milk
- 150g of frozen peas
- 350g of pasta
- 250g of ricotta cheese
- Olive oil
- 2 leeks
- 2 cloves of garlic
- 60g of Parmesan cheese
- 100ml of chicken stock
- 100ml of white wine

Directions

- Preheat the oven to 350°F and grease your baking dish.
- Then, cook the pasta in a large pan of boiling salted water, let be undercooked.
- Drain any excess water.

- Return to the saucepan and coat with a drizzle of olive oil.
- Place butter in a frying pan, fry the leeks for 10 minutes.
- Add the garlic, stock, and wine and cook for 10 minutes.
- Add the peas, cook for 30 seconds, stirring once.
- Add the leek mixture, chicken, milk, and 2/3 of the ricotta to the drained pasta.
- Let combine.
- Season with salt and pepper.
- Spoon the pasta mixture into the baking dish.
- Top with the remaining ricotta, grate over the Parmesan, and drizzle with olive oil.
- Bake for 25 minutes.
- Serve and enjoy.

Sweet leek, ricotta, and tomato lasagna

Ingredients

- 1 packet of lasagna sheets
- 4 leeks, thinly sliced
- 75g of fresh parmesan, grated
- 2 red onions, thinly sliced
- Sea salt
- 250g of spinach
- Olive oil
- 350g of ricotta
- Freshly ground black pepper
- 1-liter tomato sauce
- 125g of mozzarella ball

Directions

- Preheat your oven ready to 350°F.
- Heat a large saucepan, add a splash of olive oil when hot.
- Add the leeks together with the sliced red onions, and sweat, for 10 minutes.
- Add the chopped spinach and briefly cook until wilted down.

- Drain off any excess.
- Mix the ricotta into the leek and onion mixture.
- Season with a tiny pinch of salt and pepper.
- Spoon a quarter of the tomato sauce into the bottom of 6 individual ovenproof dishes.
- Cover with sheets of lasagna.
- Then, spread half the leek and ricotta mixture over the lasagna.
- Add the remaining tomato sauce. Repeat with all the lasagna sheets, leek and ricotta mixture, and the remaining tomato sauce.
- But finish with a layer of lasagna sheets.
- Tear the mozzarella into small pieces and dot over the top of the lasagna.
- Sprinkle with the Parmesan.
- Bake the individual lasagna for 30 minutes.
- Serve and enjoy.

Sausages with pan cooked chutney and leek mash

Ingredients

- 5cm piece of fresh ginger, grated
- 1kg of potatoes, peeled and halved
- 3 tablespoons of balsamic vinegar
- Olive oil
- 2.5cm piece cinnamon stick
- 2 leeks, sliced
- 1 handful of fresh cranberries
- 2 red onions, cut into thin wedges
- 8 pork sausages
- 200ml of milk
- Extra virgin olive oil
- 1 sprig fresh sage, leaves picked

Directions

- Begin by cooking the potatoes in simmering water for 15 minutes.
- Drain, cover and set aside.
- Add olive of oil to a separate saucepan with the leeks.

71

- Sweat gently for about 5 minutes.
- Then, add bring to the boil the milk.
- Turn off the heat, then add to the potatoes.
- Mash and season to taste. Cover and set aside.
- Preheat the grill to medium.
- Add a splash of olive oil to a frying pan over a medium heat.
- Fry the sage leaves until crisp, set aside.
- Sauté the onions for 5 minutes, add the cranberries together with the cinnamon and a splash of water.
- Let simmer for 15 minutes, stirring, until the onions are soft.
- Add the ginger together with the vinegar, cook for 30 seconds. Season.
- Place the sausages under the grill for 15 minutes, turning frequently, until cooked.
- Serve and enjoy with the chutney, mash, and sage leaves.

Slow roasted balsamic tomatoes with baby leeks and basil

Ingredients

- 12 plum tomatoes
- 200ml of balsamic vinegar
- 4 cloves garlic
- 2 tablespoons of extra virgin olive oil
- Freshly ground black pepper
- 1 handful of fresh basil
- 12 fresh bay leaves
- 12 baby leeks
- Sea salt

Directions

- Preheat the oven to 325°F.
- Score the tops of the tomatoes with a cross.
- Take an earthenware dish that the tomatoes will fit snugly into.
- Sprinkle the garlic and basil all over the bottom.
- Stand the tomatoes next to each other in the tray, on top of the garlic and basil, then push

the bay leaves well into the scores in the tomatoes, season.

- Lay the leeks on a board.
- Sprinkle generously with salt and pepper.
- Squeeze the seasoning into the mixture by pressing with a rolling pin.
- Weave the leeks in and around the tomatoes.
- Pour over the balsamic vinegar, drizzle over the olive oil.
- Let bake in the preheated oven for 1 hour.
- Remove the bay leaves.
- Serve and enjoy over pasta.

Roasted concertina squid with grilled leeks and a warm chorizo dressing

Ingredients

- 4 medium-sized squid
- Extra virgin olive oil
- 100g of chorizo sausage
- 2 cloves garlic
- 8 baby leeks
- 3 tablespoons of balsamic vinegar
- Olive oil
- Juice from one lime
- 1 sprig fresh rosemary
- 2 lemons, halved
- Sea salt
- Freshly ground black pepper
- 1 bulb fennel
- 1 radicchio, leaves separated

Directions

- Firstly, preheat a griddle pan.
- Then, preheat your oven ready to 475°F.

- Parboil the baby leeks for 3 minutes in a pan of boiling salted water.
- Drain in a colander, then let steam dry.
- Dress with some olive oil and a pinch of sea salt.
- Griddle, and cook the leek until marked with the griddle lining, add the fennel wedges, chargrill these dry on both sides until they are also marked.
- Add the radicchio leaves and dry grill to wilt.
- Put the leeks fennel and radicchio into a large bowl.
- Heat a frying pan with olive oil.
- Fry the chorizo until the fat renders out, then add the rosemary with the garlic, toss briefly and remove.
- Add the balsamic vinegar with some lemon juice to the pan, mix.
- Drizzle some olive oil over each squid, sprinkle with some salt and pepper, toss.

- Preheat an ovenproof pan with bit of olive oil, toss the reserved tentacles in the oil for 1 minute.
- Add all the squid and whack the pan in the preheated oven briefly until cooked.
- Pour the chorizo dressing over your chargrilled veggies with a squeeze of lemon juice.
- Serve and enjoy.

Roasted baby leek with thyme

Ingredients

- 2 cloves garlic
- 20 baby leeks
- 1 teaspoon of chopped fresh thyme leaves
- Olive oil
- Red wine vinegar

Directions

- Preheat your oven ready to 400°F.
- Place the leeks in a pan of boiling salted water for 3 minutes.
- Drain any excess water.
- Toss with olive oil, chopped thyme leaves, a splash of red wine vinegar, and the garlic in a bowl.
- Arrange the leeks in one layer in a baking tray.
- Let roast in the preheated oven for 10 minutes or so until golden.
- Serve and enjoy.

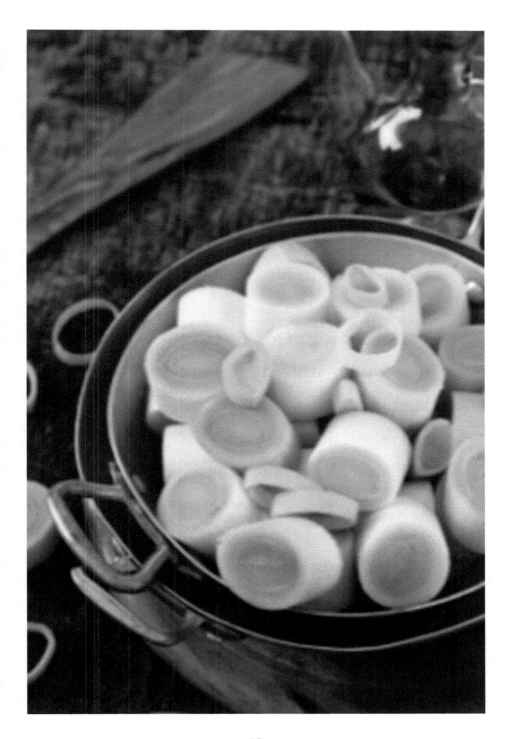

Roasted chicken breast with pancetta, leeks, and thyme

Ingredients

- Olive oil
- 1 chicken breast
- 1 pinch of sea salt
- 2 whole sprigs thyme
- 1 pinch of freshly ground black pepper
- 1 large leek
- 1 small swig of white wine
- 4 slices of pancetta

Directions

- Preheat the oven to 400°F.
- Place 1 chicken breast in a bowl.
- Add the leek, leek leaves, fresh thyme, pinch of salt, black pepper, swig of white wine, and olive oil, toss.
- Place the leek with the flavorings into the tray.
- Wrap the chicken breast in 4 slices of pancetta.
- Drizzle with olive oil, place whole thyme sprigs on top.

- Let cook for 35 minutes in the preheated.

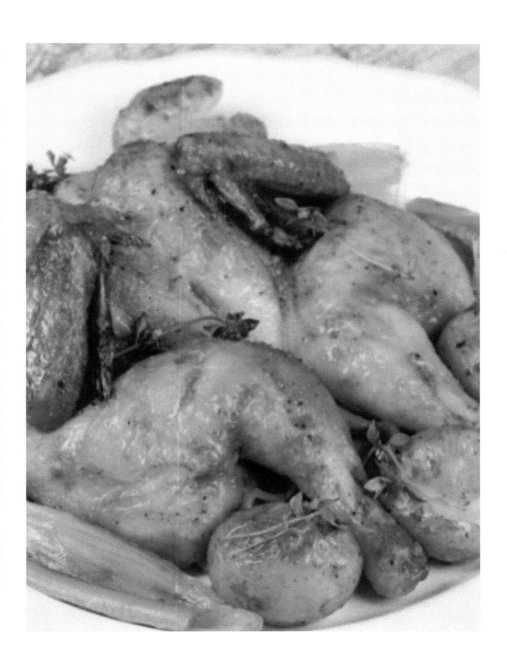

Chargrilled marinated vegetables

Ingredients

- 2 red peppers
- 1 clove garlic
- 1 large bunch of fresh basil
- 2 tablespoons of herb
- 2 yellow peppers
- 2 medium courgettes
- 1 bulb fennel
- 1 aubergine
- 8 baby leeks
- Freshly ground black pepper
- Sea salt
- Extra virgin olive oil

Directions

- Griddle pan, place all peppers on until black on all sides.
- Grill the courgette with the fennel together for 1 minute on each side.
- Transfer to a clean tea towel in one layer.

- Chargrill the aubergine slices, turn 4 times until marked.
- Transfer to the tea towel.
- Boil the baby leeks in salted water until cooked.
- Drain, then rub with bit of olive oil, and chargrill until lightly marked.
- Place all the vegetables into a large bowl.
- Bash some basil leaves in a pestle and mortar with a pinch of seasoning until a smooth pulp.
- Add about 8 tablespoons of extra virgin olive oil with vinegar.
- Pour over the vegetables and toss to coat in the basil oil. Discard the remaining basil leaves.
- Add sliced garlic to the bowl with the fennel tops.
- Give everything a good mix.
- Serve and enjoy.

Grilled fillet steak with the creamiest white beans and leeks

Ingredients

- 4 x 200g of fillet steaks
- 4 leeks
- 1 lemon
- Sea salt
- 1 small bunch of fresh thyme
- 2 cloves garlic
- Olive oil
- 1 small wineglass white wine
- Freshly ground black pepper
- 500g of tinned butter beans
- Peppery extra virgin olive oil
- 1 small handful freshly picked parsley leaves
- 1 tablespoon of fat-free natural yoghurt

Directions

- Firstly, sweat the leeks together with the thyme and garlic in a saucepan with a splash of olive oil over low heat for 20 minutes.
- Raise the heat, then add the white wine.

- Let the wine come to the boil.
- After which add the beans with a splash of water, just to almost cover the beans.
- Let simmer for 10 minutes until the beans are creamy.
- Add the parsley together with the yoghurt and extra virgin olive oil.
- Taste, and adjust the seasoning.
- Heat a griddle pan until hot, season the steaks and pat with olive oil.
- Grill a steak for 3 minutes on each side for medium-rare.
- Remove from the grill on to a dish, let rest for 5 minutes.
- Squeeze over some lemon juice and drizzle with extra virgin olive oil.
- Carve the steaks into thick slices.
- Divide the creamy beans between plates and place the steak on top
- Serve and enjoy drizzled with resting juices.

Gravadlax recipe

Ingredients

- 50g of fresh grated horseradish
- 1 big bunch of fresh dill
- 200g of raw beets
- 1 lemon
- 100g of rock salt
- 50g of demerara sugar
- 1 x 700g side of salmon
- 50ml of vodka

Directions

- Place the beets in a food processor together with sugar, vodka, salt, and dill.
- Grate in the lemon zest and add horseradish, blend to combine.
- Rub bit of the mixture on to the salmon skin, then put on a large tray, skin side down, cover completely with the mixture.
- Cover the tray tightly with Clingfilm with a weight on top.
- Place into the fridge for 36 hours.

- Once cured, unwrap the fish, pour the juices down the sink and rub salty topping.
- Pat the fillet dry, then tightly wrap in Clingfilm. Keep in the fridge until needed.
- Slice and enjoy.

Beetroot, carrot, and orange salad

Ingredients

- ½ a bunch of fresh coriander
- Olive oil
- 2 oranges
- 500g of raw beetroot
- 1 tablespoon of sesame seeds
- 750g of carrots
- Extra virgin olive oil

Directions

- Preheat the oven to 400°F.
- Parboil the carrots in a large pan of boiling salted water for 5 minutes.
- Move to a colander using a slotted spoon.
- Place in the beets and parboil for 5 minutes, then drain.
- Transfer the carrots with the beets to a large roasting tin, then, drizzle with olive oil.
- Season with sea salt and black pepper.
- Let roast for 40 minutes, or until shiny, shake the tray occasionally.

- Toast the sesame seeds over low heat until golden, tossing regularly.
- Let cool, toss with the orange zest and segments, extra virgin olive oil.
- Arrange over a large platter, scatter over the toasted sesame seeds and coriander leaves.
- Serve and enjoy.

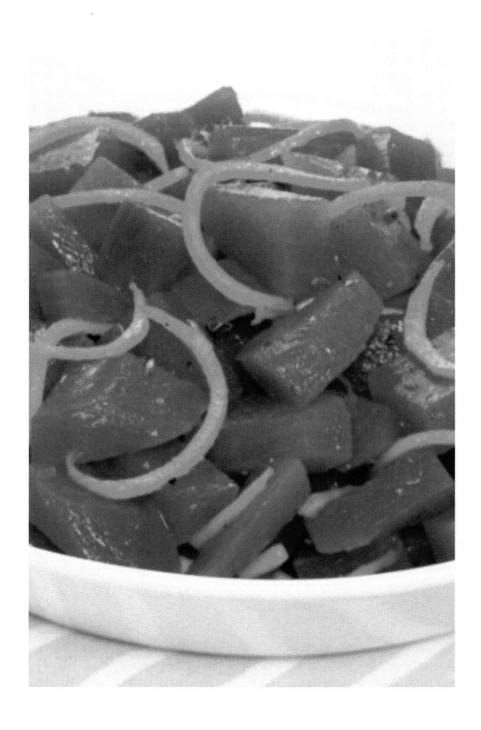

Potato rosti with beetroot horseradish

Ingredients

- 1½ teaspoons of cumin seeds
- 2 medium beetroots
- ½ a red onion
- 2 tablespoons of creamed horseradish
- 1 clove of garlic
- 2 large potatoes
- 3 tablespoons of vegetable oil

Directions

- Coarsely grate and squeeze out excess liquid from the potatoes.
- Then, combine the potatoes together with the onion, toasted cumin, and garlic in a large bowl, season.
- Shape into 4 patties with your hands.
- Heat olive oil in a pan.
- Fry the rosti over a medium-low heat for 10 minutes on each side, turning carefully.

- Combine the grated beetroot with horseradish in a bowl and serve on top of the rosti.
- Enjoy.

Beetroot nicoise salad

Ingredients

- 1 bunch of fresh mixed soft herbs
- 2 small cos lettuce
- 4 slices of sourdough bread
- 12 quail eggs
- 500g of raw mixed baby beetroots
- 1 tablespoon of red wine vinegar
- 2 teaspoons of Dijon mustard
- 1 tablespoon of baby capers
- 4 salted anchovy fillets
- 4 tablespoons of extra virgin olive oil
- 150g of fine French beans
- 100g of ripe cherry tomatoes

Directions

- Boil water in large pans.
- Place beetroots into one of the pans, keeping some for later, let boil for 10 minutes. Slice the reserved beets.
- Whisking extra virgin olive oil with vinegar, mustard, and capers.

- Season with sea salt and black pepper.
- Drain the beetroots in a colander and steam dry.
- Peel the skin and slice any larger beetroots in half.
- Transfer the beetroots to a bowl, drizzle over half the dressing, toss to coat.
- In the other pan, add the quail eggs with the French beans, let simmer for 4 minutes, then drain.
- Add the flavoring herbs to the leftover dressing, place into a salad bowl.
- Layer up the tomatoes in the salad bowl with the lettuce and anchovies, drizzle over the dressing.
- Next, tumble in the cooked and raw beetroots with the eggs and green beans.
- Scatter over the remaining herbs.
- Serve and enjoy with the sourdough.

Beetroot crisp with coriander hummus

Ingredients

- 1 teaspoon of smoked paprika
- 250g of large beetroot
- 1 lemon
- 3 sprigs of fresh thyme
- 2 tablespoons of tahini
- Olive oil
- Extra virgin olive oil
- 2 cloves of garlic
- 1 x 400g tin of chickpeas
- 50g of coriander leaves

Directions

- Preheat your oven ready to 400°F.
- Place sliced beetroots in a bowl. Toss in the thyme leaves with bit of olive oil.
- Spread on a lined baking trays, let roast for 15 minutes, let cool.
- In a blender, crush the garlic, and pour in the chickpeas with their juices.

- Add the remaining ingredients with bit of extra virgin olive oil, blend until smooth.
- Season, drizzle with extra virgin olive oil in a bowl.
- Serve and enjoy.

Roasted beetroot, red onion, and watercress salad

Ingredients

- 5 tablespoons of olive oil
- 3 tablespoons of baby caper
- 2 x 600g bunches of beetroot
- 4 red onions
- 125ml of white wine
- A few sprigs of fresh dill
- 4 tablespoons of extra virgin olive oil
- A few sprigs of fresh mint leaves
- 4 cloves of garlic
- A few sprigs of parsley leaves
- 2 x 75g bags of watercress
- 3 tablespoons of balsamic vinegar
- 1 tablespoon of Dijon mustard

Directions

- Preheat the oven to 340°F.
- Place sliced beetroots in a baking tin with 2 tablespoons of olive oil, fill the tin with water.
- Cover the dish with tin foil, let bake for 1 hour.
- Remove the beets from the tin, let cool.
- Toss the onion wedges in 2 tablespoons of the olive oil on the baking tray, season.
- Add to the oven, let roast for about 30 minutes.
- Remove, let cool.
- Rub the off the beetroot skins, cut into wedges.
- Blanch the beetroot stalks and leaves in a pan of boiling salted water for 2 minutes, drain.
- Heat the remaining tablespoon of oil in a pan over a high heat.
- Then, add the beetroot stalks and garlic and fry until the garlic is golden.
- Lower the heat to medium, pour in the wine, let cook for 10 minutes.
- Add the beetroot leaves, season, cook until wilted.

- Whisk the vinegar into the mustard, then stir in the olive oil and season to taste.
- In a large serving bowl, gently toss the roasted beetroot and red onions with the stalk mixture, chopped herbs, capers and vinaigrette, then mix with the watercress.
- Serve and enjoy.

Harvest salad

Ingredients

- 2 tablespoon of red wine vinegar
- 6 tablespoons of extra virgin olive oil
- 6 small beetroots
- 1 red onion
- 2 bulbs of fennel
- 1 teaspoon of Dijon mustard
- Olive oil
- 2 teaspoons of coriander seeds
- ½ a bunch of fresh mint
- 1 acorn squash
- ½ a bunch of fresh flat-leaf parsley
- 1 pomegranate
- 150g of feta cheese

Directions

- Preheat the oven ready to 380°F.
- Lay cut squash pieces, beetroots, fennel wedges and sliced onions in a roasting tray.
- Drizzle with a little olive oil.

- Pound the coriander seeds with a good pinch each of sea salt and black pepper.
- Sprinkle over the vegetables on the tray, toss to coat.
- Let roast for about 40 minutes, shaking halfway through. Let cool slightly.
- The, combine the vinegar together with the extra virgin olive oil, mustard, and seasoning in a small jug. Mix well.
- Dress the roasted veg while still warm so they soak up all the dressing.
- Sprinkle over the herb leaves, and reserved fennel tops.
- Add the pomegranate to the vegetables. Crumble over the feta.
- Serve and enjoy.

Roasted beetroot toast

Ingredients

- 4 slices of sourdough
- A few fresh chives
- 4 tablespoons of red wine vinegar
- 4 raw beetroots
- 5 sprigs of fresh thyme
- 2 tablespoons of creamed horseradish

Directions

- Preheat the oven to 350°F.
- Place wedges of beetroot in a roasting tray.
- Add the vinegar together with the thyme and 4 tablespoons of water, toss to coat.
- Cover with tin foil, then let roast for 45 minutes.
- Toast the bread and spread with the horseradish topping with the roasted beetroot.
- Serve and enjoy.

Warm potato, herring, beetroot and apple salad

Ingredients

- 4 tablespoons of olive oil
- 200g of beetroot
- 2 tablespoons of red wine vinegar
- 1 pinch of granulated sugar
- 500g of Ratte potatoes
- A few fresh chives
- 1 small apple
- 1 lug of sparkling water
- 2 marinated herring fillets
- ½ tablespoon of Dijon mustard

Directions

- For the vinaigrette, combine the Dijon mustard together with the olive oil, red wine vinegar, and sugar in a bowl.
- Season with sea salt and black pepper, then whisk to blend.
- Add the sparkling water to loosen the mixture, then whisk.

- Cook the beetroot in a pan of boiling salted water for 45 minutes.
- In another separate pan of boiling salted water, cook unpeeled potatoes for 20 minutes. Drain in a colander, then slice warm.
- Drain and allow the beetroot to cool slightly, then slice.
- Divide the potato, beetroot, apple slices and herring fillets among 4 serving plates.
- Drizzle over the vinaigrette, chop and scatter over the chives.
- Serve and enjoy with warm potatoes.

Beetroot dip

Ingredients

- 4 vac-packed beetroot
- 1 tablespoon of horseradish
- Rye bread
- 1 teaspoon of caraway seeds
- 3 sprigs of fresh thyme
- 3 tablespoons of crème fraiche

Directions

- Pick the thyme leaves, and blend all the ingredients in a food processor.
- Season with sea salt and black pepper.
- Serve and enjoy with rye bread.

Beetroot, almond, and ricotta

Ingredients

- 2 tablespoons of ground almonds
- 2 tablespoons of ricotta cheese
- Vac-packed cooked beetroot

Directions

- Place the beetroot in a blender.
- Add the ground almonds together with the ricotta cheese to the blender, a purée.
- Adjust thickness with water.
- Serve and enjoy.

Chili pickled sweet and sour beets

Ingredients

- 3 fresh red chillies
- 100ml of balsamic vinegar
- 1 tablespoon coriander seeds
- 400ml of white wine vinegar
- 200g of golden caster sugar
- 1/2 lemon
- 1.5 kg of beetroots

Directions

- Place the beets in a pan of salted water and bring to the boil.
- Let simmer for 30 minutes until cooked, then drain. Let cool.
- Add the vinegars together with the sugar in a separate pan.
- Add halved chilies to the pan with a squeeze of lemon juice, coriander seeds, and a pinch of sea salt, over a high heat.
- Bring to the boil, stirring until the sugar is dissolved.

- Spoon the beets into jars, pour the pickling liquid on top.
- Add a chili to each jar, seal, infuse for few days
- Serve and enjoy.

Lightning Source UK Ltd.
Milton Keynes UK
UKHW020749030621
384855UK00001B/70